DEDICATION

I dedicate this book to my kids.

Aly, Andy, Calvin, I truly do have the greatest daughter and sons in the world.

I pray the situations you face in life because of this illness make you strong, understanding, caring adults.

CONTENTS

ACKNOWLEDGMENTS

Thank you Mikey for standing behind me and my endless list of half-finished projects. Thank you for supporting my ideas, no matter how crazy they may seem. Soul-mates.

Vikki, thank you for removing the southern drawl and bad grammar from my writing. I know you never dreamed of what has become when you agreed to edit for me. Our friendship means the world to me.

And finally,

Aly, Andy, Calvin. Thank you for inspiring me to write this book. As Calvin would say, "I love you Buddy!" All of this is for you three.

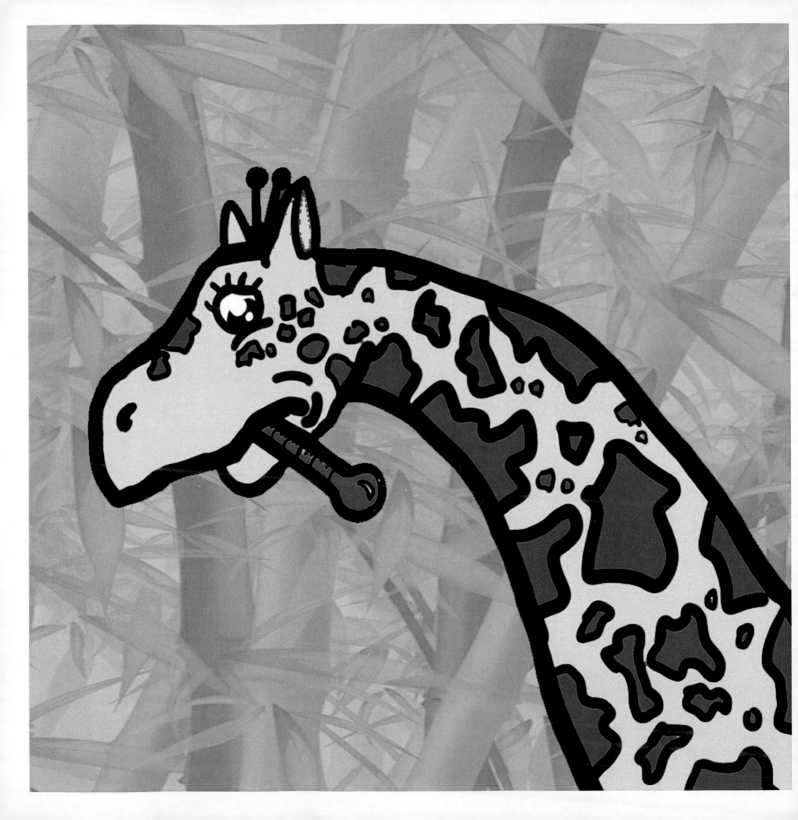

One day my mommy started feeling ill.

She went to the doctor, and he did a bunch of tests. The tests said my Mommy had Multiple Sclerosis, but the doctor called it MS. I was really scared, but Mommy told me she was going to be ok.

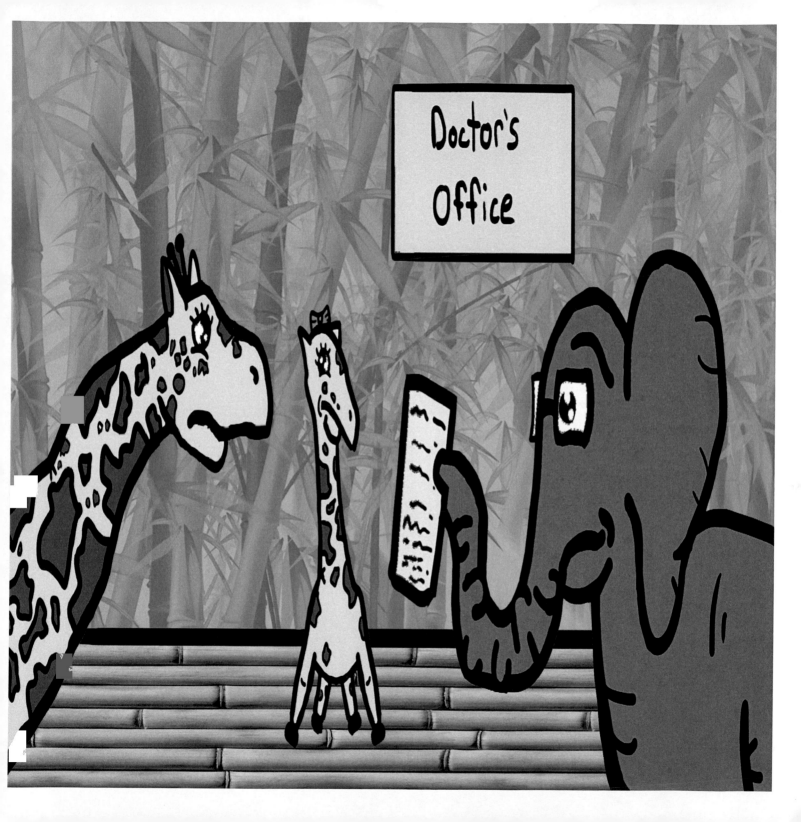

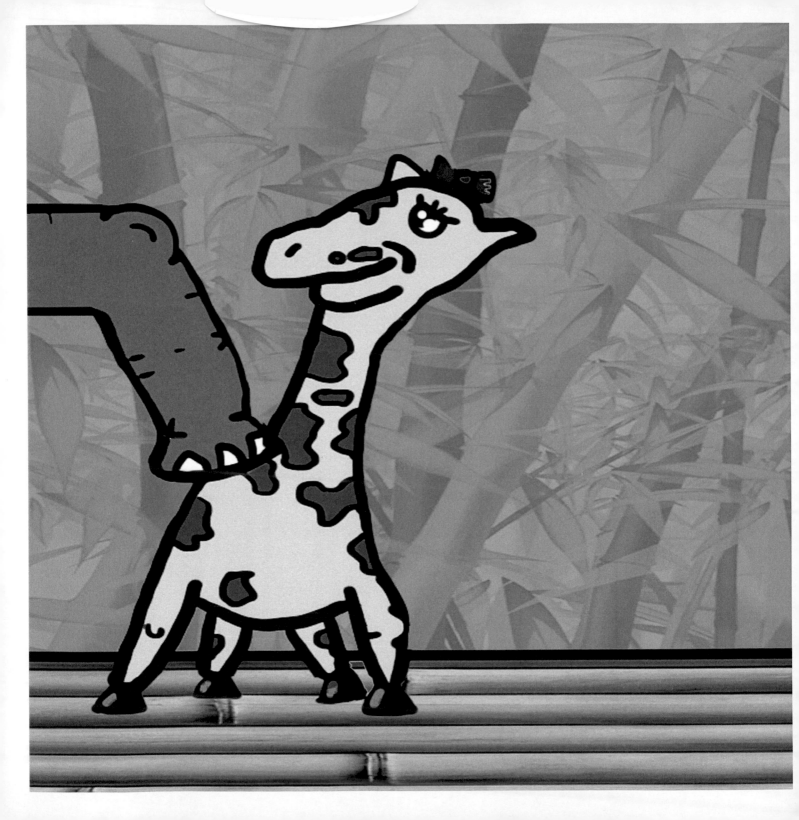

The doctor explained that I could help Mommy out by helping her around the house and by being on my best behavior, so Mommy would not get upset.

We went home and researched MS on Mommy's computer. It said MS happens when the messages from her body to her brain get messed up because they are traveling on a bumpy road.

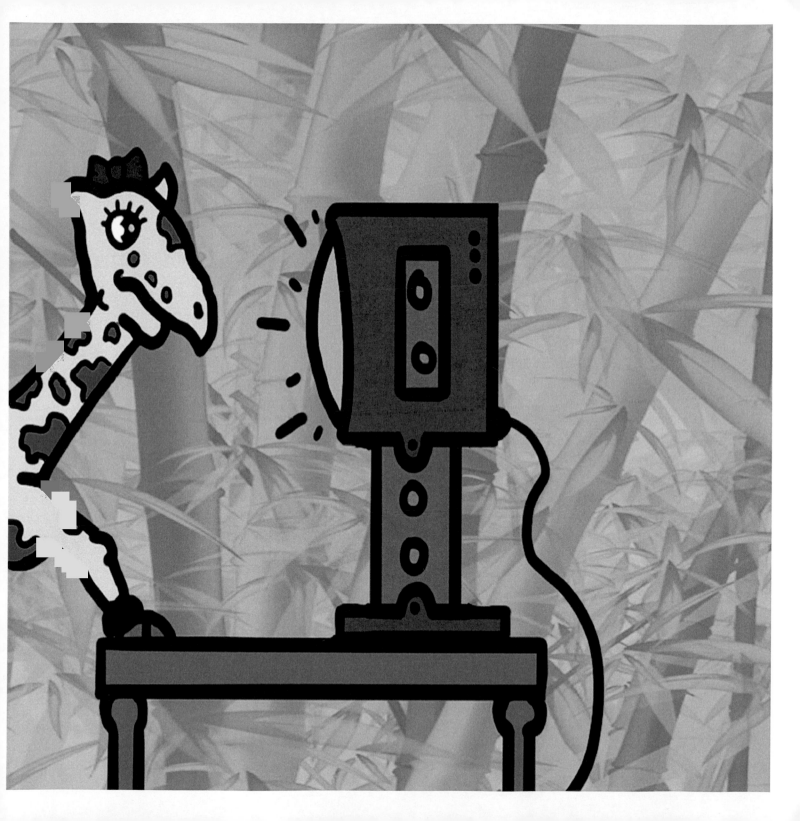

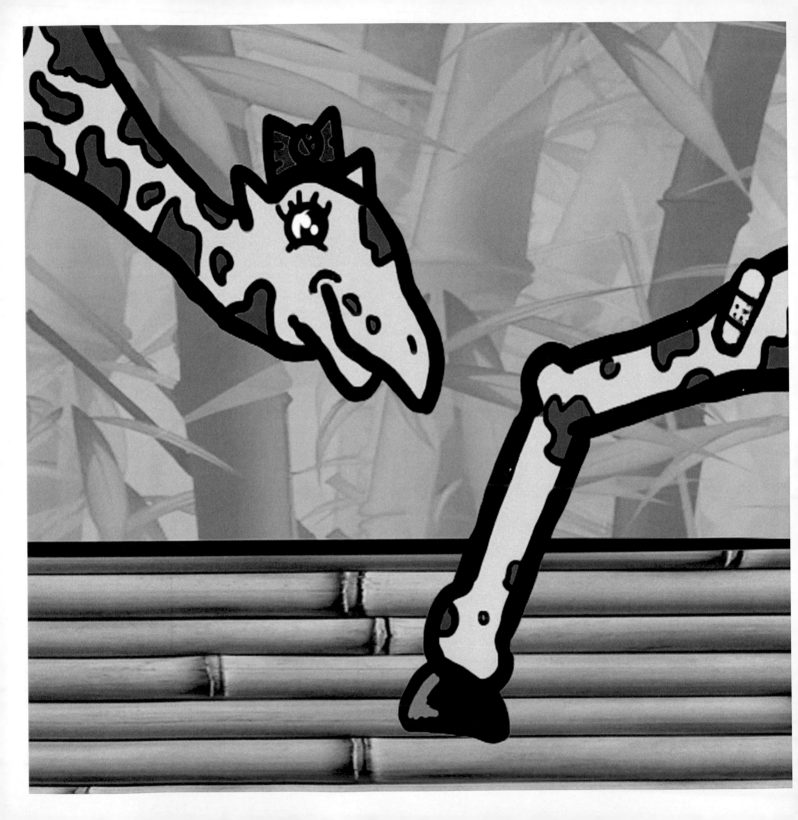

Mommy takes medication that helps her stay well. She uses a small needle to put the medication in her leg. Sometimes she lets me put the bandage on when she finishes.

Sometimes Mommy is really tired and her body feels funny. I help her by keeping my room clean and being extra quiet while she rests.

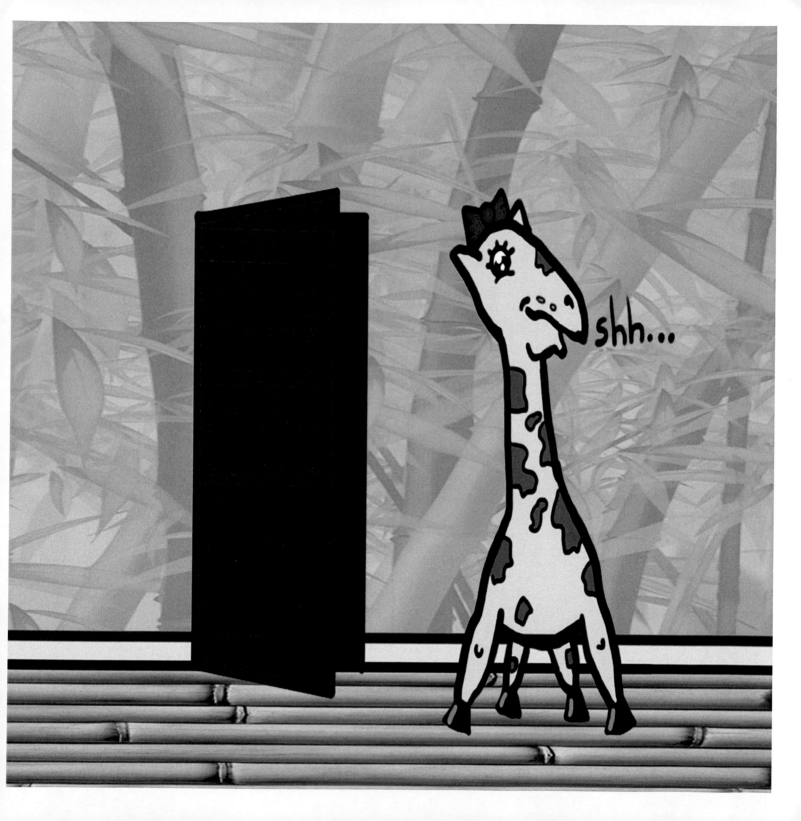

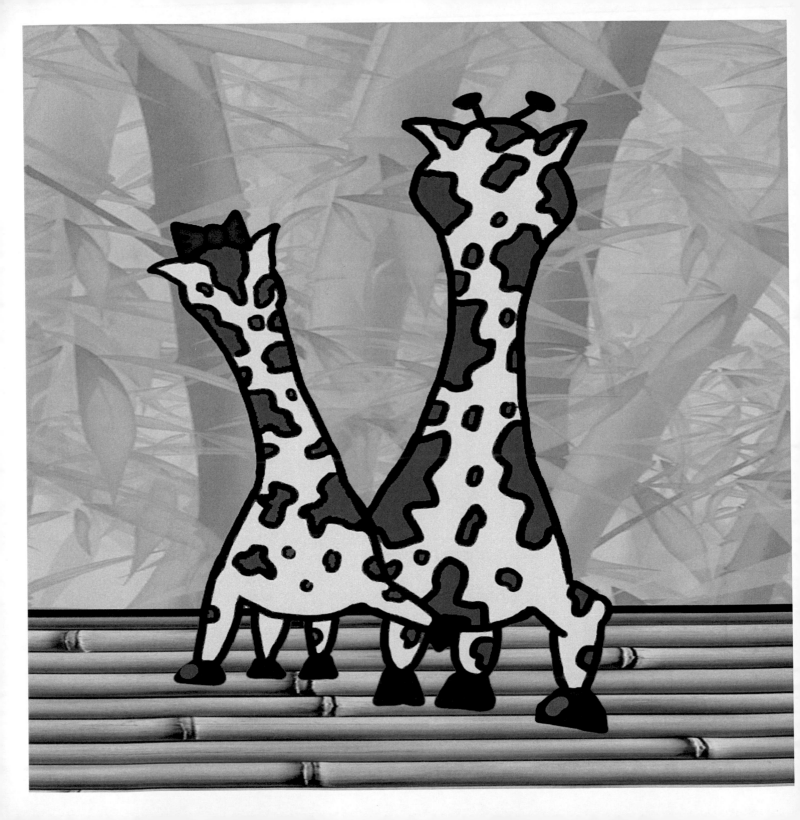

Sometimes Mommy has trouble walking, so I help her balance when we walk around.

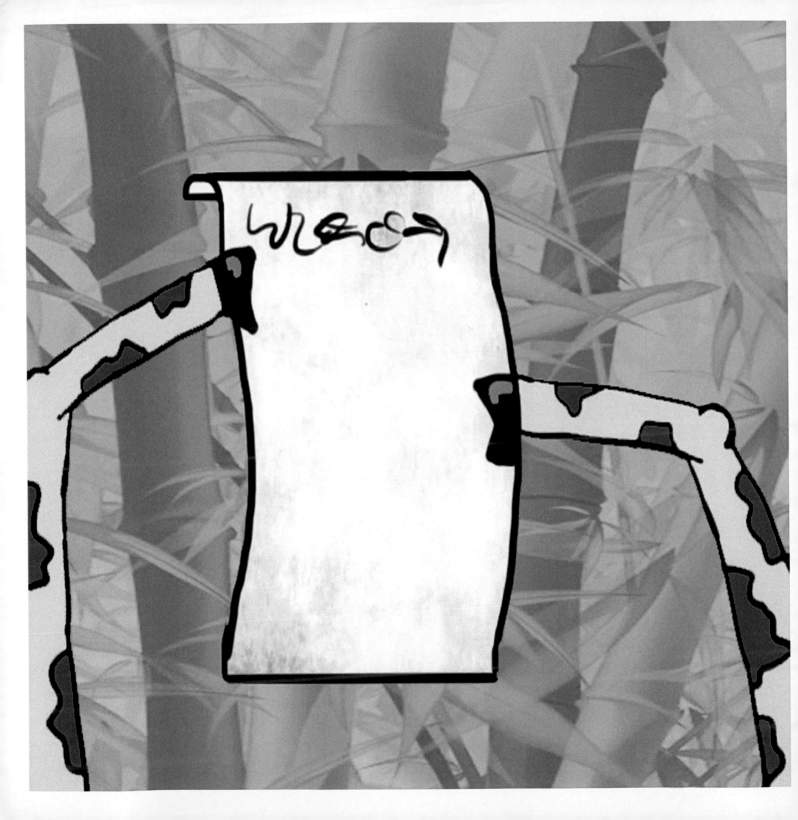

Sometimes Mommy's eyes act funny. She sees 2 of everything! I help her read the words when she cannot.

Some days Mommy feels great and takes me to the park. When it is hot, she tries to stay cool by wearing a vest with ice in it. The heat can make Mommy get sick.

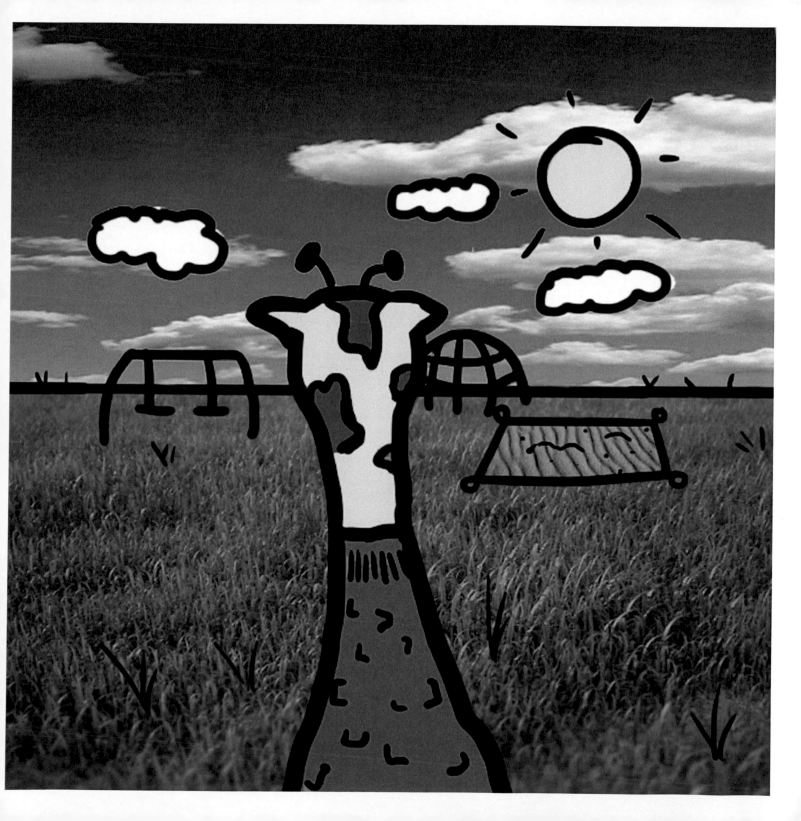

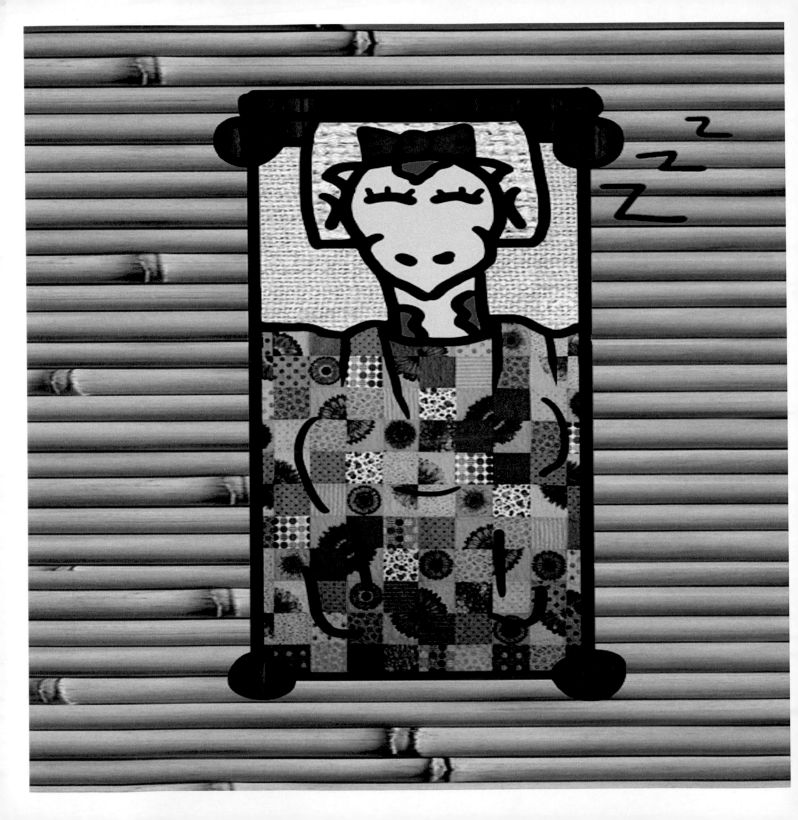

Before I go to sleep, Mommy tucks me in and says "I am so happy I have such an amazing daughter, thank you for helping me."

When I grow up, I want to help people with MS, like my Mommy.

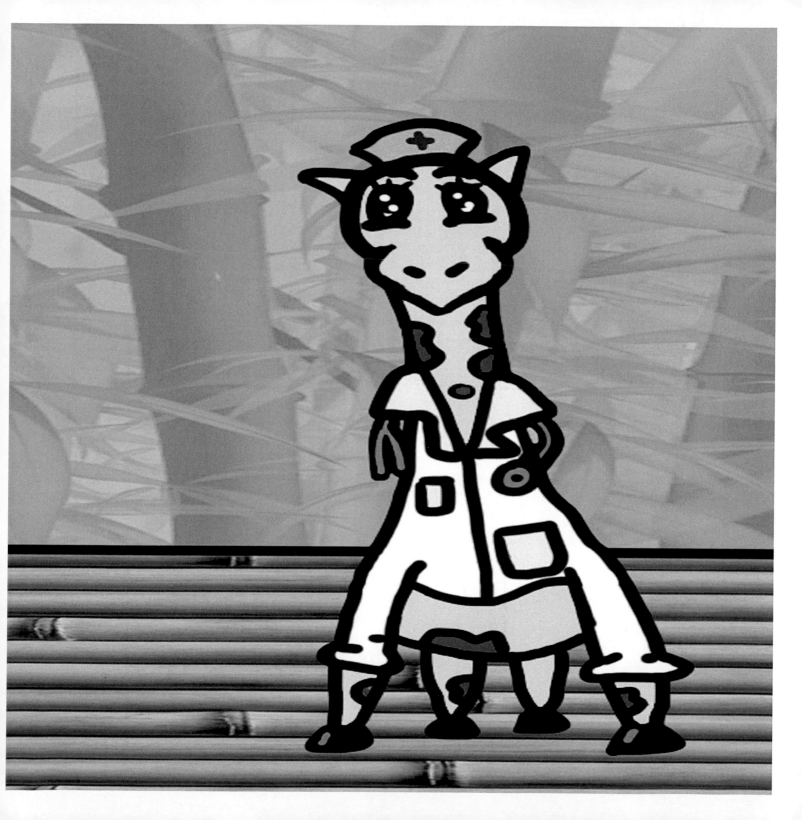

Kid Friendly Glossary and Tips

This glossary is meant to give you ideas on how to describe the various objects and symptoms associated with Multiple Sclerosis. This is not a one sized fit all approach, so use your imagination and creativity when describing something to your children. Tell the truth, but keep it age/maturity appropriate. Remember, it never hurts to paint something in a positive light.

Acute
Something that happens fast, but doesn't last long.

Assistance Devices
If referring to something specific, it is best to call it by name. Otherwise explaining the object and specific function can help children understand and ease any fears associated with it.

Autoimmune Disease
Autoimmune diseases cause problems with the nervous system, the part of the body that carries messages around the body.

Brain
The organ that is in your head, behind your eyes. It controls what the body does.

Catheter
A straw like tube that helps someone use the bathroom when they need to.

Chronic
Opposite of Acute: Something that lasts a long time, sometimes forever.

Cognition
The way the brain works.

Coordination
When parts of the body work together to make something happen, such as walking.

Demyelination
Losing the outer covering of the nervous system.

Disability
The lack of ability to do something as well as and in the amount of time other people can do it.

Exacerbation
An "episode" or "situation" when symptoms appear or get worse.

Gene
A small part of the body that has the instructions to create other things in the body.

Immune System
The system that identifies bad or damaged things and attempts to make them go away.

Impairment
The loss of the ability to do something in the same way as before.

Inflammation
What parts of the body does when injury happens.

Intravenous
In a vein, the lines that you can see under the skin.

Lesion
A damaged area.

MRI
A tool used to look inside the body.

Myelin
A soft, white lining on the outside of the nervous system.

Nerve
The path in which messages travel around the body.

Nervous System
The brain, the spinal cord, and all the nerves in the body.

Neurologist
A doctor who finds and helps with nervous system illnesses.

Optic Neuritis
The nerves that control the eye inflame, causing issues with the eye and the way you see.

Paralysis
Not being able to move a part of the body.

Plaque
An area of the nervous system that is inflamed.

Prognosis
Prediction of the future of the illness.

Rehabilitation
Practicing something to help improve everyday functions.

Remission
Period of time when decreasing or disappearing symptoms occur.

Sclerosis
Hardening of tissue in the body.

Sensory
How your body understands various things such as pain, smell, taste, temperature, vision, hearing, and speech.

Spasticity
When the body resists movement.

Symptom
A problem or complaint related to an issue.

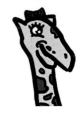

Gail's Chore Chart- Month

Name: _____ **Month:** _____

Sunday	Monday	Tuesday	Wednesday	Thursday	Friday	Saturday

(Printable charts available for download at www.MyMommyHasMS.com)

ABOUT THE AUTHOR

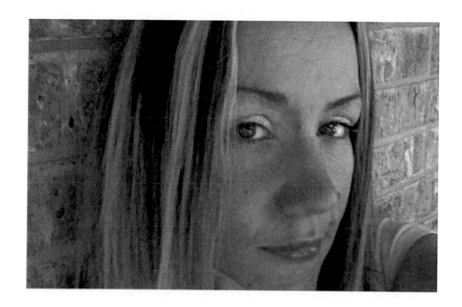

Rebecca Clary was diagnosed with Multiple Sclerosis November 2008 after an episode sitting in a store parking lot convinced her she should stop driving until she got her eyes checked. 2 days later she sat in an emergency room with a diagnosis. She had 2 children at the time, an 18 month old and a 9 month old, and gave birth to her 3rd child 16 months after diagnosis. Shocked by the lack of support groups for parents with MS, she founded the Parenting With MS Support Group in 2009.

Made in the USA
San Bernardino, CA
09 August 2015